Dedication

I dedicate this book to each and everyone who trusted in me to help them to get their lives back. I am grateful to be chosen to do this work. Your successes are my greatest reward.

I would like to introduce you to one of my most INSPIRING clients, Mike Ratcliffe. Mike came to me in 2016 suffering from constant pain in his neck and lower back. He had been in pain management for 3 years prior to meeting me. He was depressed and felt as if he couldn't go on living in pain. Mike's case was different from my other clients for one very simple reason. Mike has been living with cerebral palsy since birth and has very little, if not, zero control over the right side of his body. He spends most of his days in a power scooter since he lost his strength to walk as a child. However, that this is where Mike's remarkable story begins.

If you were to ask Mike if he were handicapped, he would say the same thing each time, "I don't know the meaning of the word!" This man had such a will to live a normal life and his condition never stopped him from doing so. Mike had a van built especially for him, so he could load his scooter into it. Once he gets inside, then it's off to the driver's seat. Nothing stops him from getting where he wants to go! However, his story doesn't stop there. Mike is a success everywhere else in his life. He is partnered with his mother with successful their realty team. They are #1 in their office and #2 in their company.

Mike has always been in-charge of his own destiny and never gave up on anything. He loves to swim, he's been repelling down huge cliffsides, and even has been skydiving! Most importantly, he is a great son, and a greater husband. His desire to live life to the fullest has helped him to create a life full of health, wealth, and happiness. So, you can imagine how this pain was taking that all away from him. I knew upon meeting Mike that the job meant so much more for him and I worked tirelessly until I got him some relief. Over the next 2 months, I was able to get his body the relief that he prayed for from this powerful work. This is proof that EVERY- BODY can accept this work in a powerful way.

Mikey, the world needs more INSPRING people like you. That is why I am sharing your story with the world. It has been an honor to help guide you back to happiness. Thank you for your trust and friendship.

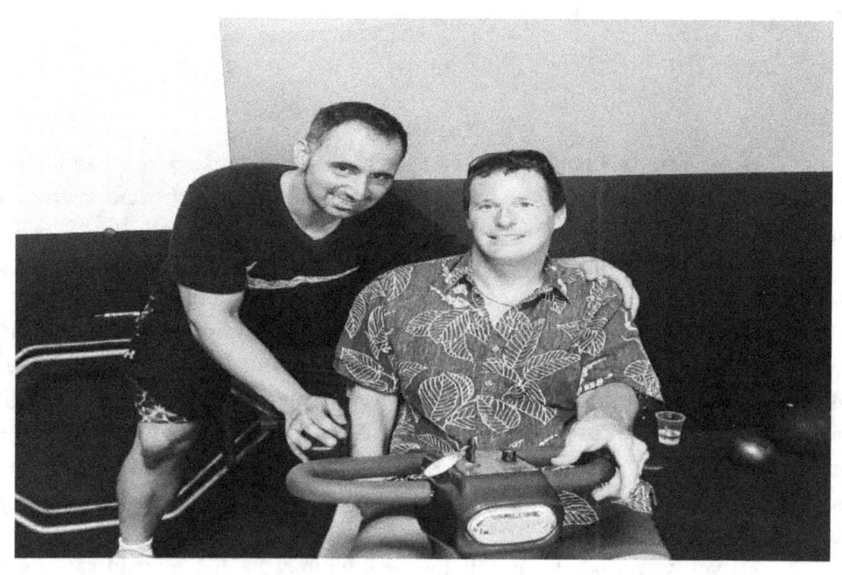

Mike Ratcliffe and Neil J. Denaut II

Foreword

This book is INSPIRED by my quest for finding solutions to my personal training clients' pains.

It was my job, then it became my purpose. Chances are that it was my purpose all along.

What if I told you that I could decompress all the muscles in someone's lumbar and sacral spine region in as little as 1 hour?

Skeptical? I'd be, but I wouldn't judge my book by its cover. Otherwise, I would not have found the most incredible solutions for my clients' pains. It's all here and it needs to be shared.

Let's put an end to chronic pain and stop the need for pain medications. Once neuromuscular balance is restored to all your muscles, then your body will begin to stop hurting itself, and start to heal.

I have over 21 years of practice looking for the best ways to help others in pain. However, the last 7 years have shown the most consistent results of my career (40,000+ practice hours). Why? Because this work has allowed me to help at least 90% of my clients, achieve at least 90% of their strength/mobility back, and in as little as 4 hours. This may not be the only way to help the body to heal, but those numbers are staggering.

My goal is to educate, enlighten, and change the world of Fitness with these principles.

The "Denaut Muscular Re-calibration System" is the missing link in Personal Training, Fitness Programming, and throughout the Physical re-habilitation world.

I hope that you enjoy my work and you use it to help EVERYONE around the world!

We are the primary solution to the physical prosperity of others. We owe it to them, to give them the BEST results possible!

ABOUT THE AUTHOR

Neil J. Denaut II began his fitness career after successfully losing 62 lbs. at the age of 19. His results drove him to learn more about strength training, nutrition, and the body. After receiving his B.A. in Psychology from Purchase College (Purchase, NY), his life turned towards the gym, and he began helping others to change their lives through fitness full-time.

Neil took a big interest in special populations like seniors. He grew up helping his grandmother out with walking and other physical activities. He wanted to do more for her, so he took courses from the companies that certified him, and went right to work. Neil worked with his grandmother for several months from a wheel chair and saw strength improvements all around. Unfortunately, it was too soon in his career to learn the powerful principles in this book, or he would have been able to do more for her. That's why his work means so much to him and helping others that needed a lot of physical help soon became his favorite type of client.

Neil has held Certifications in Personal Training for over 17 years with top fitness organizations such as AFAA and NASM. His other specialty training includes:

- Corrective Exercise Specialist (2007)
- Special Populations: Pre/post-natal, Youth, & Seniors (2007)
- Youth and Adult Athletic Conditioning via. Under Armour and IMG Academies (2010)
- Over 100 hours of Mentorship with Master Body Worker, and Master Resistance Stretching trainer Carla McEwan (2011)
- Ki-Hara Resistance Stretching Level II (2012)
- Fascia Buzz Active Release Protocol (2013)
- Neuromuscular Re-programming w/ Carla McEwan (2017)

In 2014, Neil moved his family from his lifelong home in New York, to San Diego, California so he could bring this work to the center of the Fitness Industry. He knew that moving there was where he had to be to see his DREAM come true. He has never looked back.

Neil also has served on legal teams as an expert witness in personal injury cases and has taught audiences as far as China. This is his global mission and it's just the beginning!

Table of Contents:

My Mission

I began my journey in Fitness back in early 1999. I made the decision to make a change in my body. I spent most of my childhood being overweight and not very athletic. My step-dad Rob showed me how to train and told me what I needed to do to change my body. I faithfully jumped into this new way of doing things and within 6 months, I lost 62 pounds. I knew immediately that I had crossed a great point of no return. I had acquired the knowledge that allowed me to finally be successful in my fitness and it INSPIRED me to teach others that wanted to change their own physical fitness.

I had finally made a dream come true! That time it was one of the happiest stages of my life. So much so, that I needed to share it with everyone. It was as if I unlocked myself and truly began living. I was happier in every part of my life. I was confident, friendlier, and it was the best that I had ever felt in my entire life. I believe that everyone should feel this type of empowerment and I wanted to be the bridge for them to get there.

I began dragging my friends to my basement gym and almost forcing them to workout. Other people began asking me for help and I obliged. I began writing up Personal Training programs and teaching them how to do the work. It happened faster than I expected, and I embraced every part of it. I began to try new gyms out, new workouts, and learn more about Fitness. My primary goals as a young 20-year-old were typical for back then, stay lean, get strong, and to look like Arnold Schwarzenegger.

After College, I finally took the next step and became a full-time Fitness Professional. I was going to help EVERYONE lose weight exactly like I did! I was so excited!! That's when I quickly began to realize that it was not going to be so clear cut and easy for everyone.

I began working with a different population of clients as I started working full-time. Most of my clients were in their early 40's to mid 50's and spent their days stuck at a desk or in a car. This meant that there were now a few more obstacles to navigate around before kicking their butts with exercise. A lot of people had physical limitations that prevented them from doing any of the exercises that I wanted them to do... This troubled me for a few reasons.

1. How can I help these people reach their goals if they couldn't work out?
2. What if I hurt them more?
3. I didn't really know any more exercises so, I had to do something with them if I were to keep them as a client.
4. These people came to me for help and it was my job as a Fitness Professional to find the solutions that would help to move them forward.

I personally have had some minor injuries working out and was able to rehab myself. I also had the experience recovering from a fractured pelvis that I sustained in a car accident back in '99. I believed that people could recover on their own, however, I lacked the experience with other injuries like herniated discs, knees, and neck to have any type of familiarity or personal experience with them. The best solution that I had at that point was to recommend them to their personal Dr.

Before I continue I just want to make one thing clear: I firmly believe in Doctors and their passion for helping others.

I soon learned however, that the healthcare system had a few "gaps" in its ability to thoroughly help those with injuries. There seemed to be a total disconnect with the injured, their doctor, the insurance companies, and the treatment of the injury. The current understanding of strength rehabilitation is based on correcting symptoms. However, any injury that shows up is a systematic failure. Pain and/or damage is due to excessive mechanical overleveraging of the body. Those systems must be re-calibrated so we can restore full function to the body without pain. We must determine the root cause.

Most people tend to get injured because of a physically overwhelming and/or unhealthy lifestyle. My scope as a Fitness professional was to provide my clients with short and long-term solutions to their overall physical health. Moreover, it seemed that my clients were not achieving the success they were looking for with their injuries elsewhere. As a Fitness professional, I was more available to my clients more than any other healthcare professional. That presented a big opportunity and a big responsibility for me to dramatically change someone's life.

Fitness professionals work closer and more frequently with their clients more than other health professionals. Particularly, as Personal Trainers, we have the avenue to provide the GREATEST IMPACT on the wellness of others. Your clients come to you for what they want, and you must evaluate what they need to maximize their success in reaching their goals. Soon thereafter, the relationship becomes one of a mentor, coach, and a friend.

My success in helping my clients' pain determined my success as a trainer and our work together was the key element that brought them results. Your success as a trainer will be determined by the results that your work provides. A client's recovery and prosperity are an everyday process and their program should be addressed that way. They need to be led. We aren't just working on swapping out one physique for a new one. We are educating, coaching, inspiring, and supporting their journey. Lifestyle changes don't just change overnight, however, they need to take precedent in the lives of our clients. Part of our job is to make it a priority for them to make to adjustments in their daily activities, keeping them accountable, and make tools available that will reinforce the new education to our clients' new lifestyle. They are making a transformation much like the one that I had. It's just that everyone needs their own specific adjustments and that is why they hired you! This is where the personal part makes the biggest IMPACT in their journey.

Here is what my typical injured client may say: "I went to see so and so, but I'm still in pain or it got worse."

Why did this happen? At first, I felt like other professionals were keeping a big secret but they're not. The truth is that there are just many variables the affect how well we can recover from an injury. Most health professionals have a few set of tools to use for jobs that may require different or better tools. It is also more likely medical professional can only interact with you for a very limiting amount of time. The insurance companies tie their hands with what they will approve and pay for, how much of their time they are willing to pay them for, and it limits a lot of other health professionals from giving their patients the solutions that they need.

How do we fix it? We do it by elevating ourselves professionally. Fitness coaches spend more time with their clients than any other professional, have far more influence in their daily lives, and can provide them with a wide variety of the most effective solutions possible. Furthermore, it is our professional responsibility to lead them down the path of restoration in many facets, not just to make them sweaty.

My entire career has been based from this ideology. My unrelenting desire to provide the greatest solutions to my clients has led me to the answers that will provide your clients physical results beyond anyone's wildest dreams.

I found the game changing answers in the power of eccentric muscle stretching (EMS). As soon as I incorporated this tool into my own system for training clients, their results skyrocketed! I took that body of work and formulated what I call, "The Denaut Muscular Re-Calibration System." By using eccentric based muscle stretching (EMS), it gives us the power to immediately lengthen muscle while directly communicating with the brain. We then stretch muscle group pairs one at a time and in the correct sequences. As a result, the brain then re-calibrates your entire body to accommodate the new length-tension relationship EVERYWHERE. The moment I inserted this principle into my corrective exercise system it created an *IMMEDIATE IMPACT*. Furthermore, the results occurred up to 10 times faster than the previous methods did, and it elevated their success in every program goal that we set.

Why? Because this is the missing piece in all Fitness programming. We focus on what happens when we overload a muscle, but we almost never program for the opposite. We may acknowledge it, but it is always our secondary focus. Fitness programs should also be designed with a huge focus on eccentric muscle contraction stretching. It changes EVERYTHING about our bodies, range of motion, flexibility, and strength. You will see the body unwind right before our eyes and it last longer than any other approach!

This book is going to explain what it is, how to use it in ALL your workouts, and how it will be the answer to your clients' exercise obstacles.

This is the way that the body works! Plain and simple... It *MUST* be utilized!!

The Body Unfolded

Our body was designed to fluctuate with the imperfect environment. The world was not created flat nor with sophisticated footwear. The body was designed to absorb and displace shock as we move through life. It is designed to adapt to any environment. The very design is perfect, and its sophistication is second to none. Everything about it is finely tuned with the ability to adapt instantaneously to any situation. Furthermore, we have the greatest supercomputer on Earth (our brain) to constantly monitor all activity. It will adapt to our favored movement patterns all while keeping the body in its structural integrity.

Counter-balancing is always happening. Without counter balancing our muscles, then as we moved we would fall over or worse, we would break something. Moreover, I would like to remind you that the body is constantly in rotation. This means that every movement involves reaching across the body and at the same time, has a counter balancing torso rotation. Furthermore, our limbs (arms/leg) systematically rotate as they bend and stretch. Essentially, our bodies twist back and forth like a towel as we move in any direction. We are single side dominant being. We most likely use one side of the body over the other. This has a consequence. Over time we get wrapped in a rotated state. Now your relaxed or "neutral posture" has a twisted musculature foundation, and adding new training or information will be built on top of your twisted foundation. This will happen to all of us somehow. It is our job to identify it, correct it, and educate our clients about it. If you wanted to straighten the leaning tower of Pisa, would you just build it to lean in the opposite direction? No, you correct the foundation and the same should apply for ANY structure.

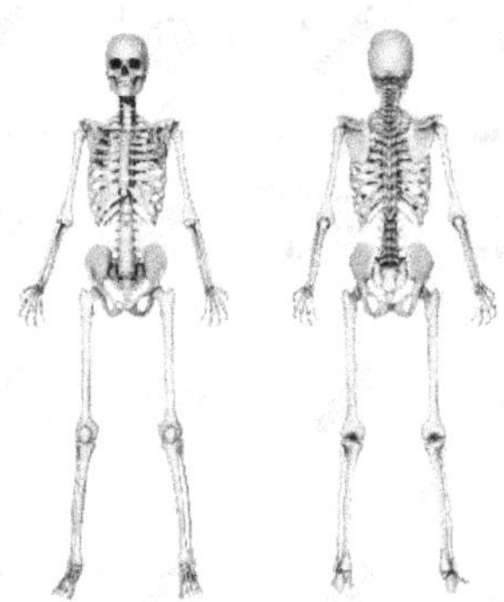

(Neutral Skeleton)

Without proper re-calibrating of the body through exercise or therapy, it will remain in the favored rotation indefinitely. Over time the musculature compresses, our skeleton becomes restricted in its ability to relax, and damage occurs. This is how the body systematically creates pain/trauma. Most approaches treat symptoms and not the systems. Your body is breaking down somewhere due to a system that is programmed to move the body when it is extremely over-leverage. Therefore, just treating the site of trauma is that it will not correct the problem. The systems must be re-calibrated to fully restore function and eliminate the problem completely.

Imagine this: Your right hip is your favorite side (dominant). Naturally, you begin all movement with your right arm moving towards the left side of the body. You aren't just reaching your arm, however, you are also creating a spiral effect in your musculature, and it ends at the right hip. Imagine the twisted towel: If you begin twisting from the upper right-hand corner towards the midline, then the lower left will immediately twist to counter-balance the upper right and ends at the right hip. As the body becomes tighter it gets stuck in rotation, thus keeping the body imbalanced all over. Eventually, it locks the right hip into in externally rotated position (or towards your dominant side, barring outlying circumstances like accidental trauma or disease). That is just one series of muscles. We also must consider how the opposing set of muscles are affected. So, what happens to the opposing muscles that are opposing the primary movement?

Most people are right handed so typically the left side chain rotation counterbalances rotation and movements that originate from the right side. The left side must follow the right and counter-balance. This means that it will adjust the tension relationship in the hip muscles, as well as in the thigh and leg muscles, to support the movement. Moreover, this also directly influences the upper body.

Yes, the left shoulder will begin tightening to towards the right hip and the left shoulder must follow the right shoulder because they are connected. Like I said, picture a twisted towel. This is a matter of mechanics, as well as, physiology. It is mechanically impossible to not have this occur. Remember, this is the perfect design of the body to adapt accordingly. It must happen. Now the neuro-musculo-skeletal system runs an adapted movement program and correcting one part of one muscle group cannot fully restore anyone's body. It may make some progress over time, however, that is too much work and still may never make it close to balanced. It just becomes more tolerable. We need systematic changes to correct symptoms.

The Facts About Surgery

Surgery corrects symptoms, yet it rarely corrects the root cause. For example, tearing a knee ligament is not because you were dealt a bad knee in your DNA. The ligament tear typically occurs because of improper muscle balances and faulty mechanics. The excessive wear and vulnerability at the knees creates trauma. We can repair the damage, however, systematically your body is showing up in the old pattern with a repaired ligament. Spinal injury, joint, and or muscle injury are almost ALWAYS mechanical damage due to poor neuro-musculo-skeletal efficiency. Do you know someone that had surgery and it still in pain? That's why. They fixed the symptom and did not correct the systems or root cause. Muscular re-calibration can prolong, and/or keep us from surgery altogether. I've seen many people that were told that they had no hope get back to life pain free.

The lower back is one of the most prominent ailments that people see their Dr.s for Back pain and it is a $90 Billion industry. The truth is that the majority of lower back injuries are correctable before they happen, and even after trauma occurs. Remember, pain is a symptom and it can be relieved. The problem is that most approaches use simple tactics that only approach the sight of pain. The fact is that your internal and external core are virtually tearing your spine apart. The approach that you will read about in this book effects the entire kinetic chain. As we get the body closer to efficiency, it will give us the access we need to address the internal musculature and release the problem.

The Hip bone is Connected to the Thigh Bone

I've heard so many arguments over time about what the right way to train a client is, what the wrong thing to do is, and how this exercise trend caused x,y,z. The first thing that ANY Personal Trainer/Strength Coach learns is the concept of Neuro-musculo-skeletal efficiency. If you don't know what this means, and you are an active Fitness Pro, then you have failed the exam. Please go directly to summer school. The right way to build any structure is with a solid and precise foundation.

If you are a Fitness pro and "sort-of" program for this, or do it with some clients, then you it's time for a shift in the way that you're thinking and step your game up.

As for everyone else, if you practice this principle in every workout that you design, then my hats off to you. You are likely to be significantly more successful than most of the industry.

Fitness professionals listen closely. I am going to present to you the most profound principle that is going to change EVERYTHING about your programming and it's going to be extremely simple.

> "Muscles can only truly become elongated/stretched while under their own tension (during the eccentric phase of contraction)."

What does that mean? It means that a muscle can and will become longer (aka less tight), if it is pulled apart while it is contracting. BOOM! Oh, but wait, there is more!

Once this change occurs several things happen in our bodies.

1. Our brain recognizes the changes in the muscle's length and it then re-calibrates everything else in the body to support it (just as it did when the muscle shortened).
2. Muscle that has been weakened or inhibited by another tight muscle begins to restore its ability to fire and do work.
3. Tight muscles lengthen, thus becoming stronger due to the increase its contraction length.
4. Our joints become less stressed
5. Our posture becomes less distorted
6. We can generate more power and strength with more efficient muscles
7. Our balance improves

And the list goes on.........

This does not just happen all within one single stretch, however, when it is continually applied, and it is done in the proper sequence, it then reverses the tension from your activities of daily life. Just 1 hour of a hands-on muscle re-calibration session can take someone with long term back pain to squatting at 90 degrees depth without pain, and it lasts! We can make changes happen immediately if we tap into our neuromuscular system the right way and this system will teach you how to do it.

This is how the body stretches with every movement. The eccentric phase of muscle contraction stretches the muscle open with help of the opposing muscle. However, once the muscle is extremely tight, its opposing partner cannot contract enough to fully lengthen/stretch its partner. Once this relationship changes, so does every other muscle group in the body. Over time, pain or damage can occur in a muscle or joint. To correct it, you will also correct the other muscle groups too and it is very likely that you must restore other muscle groups before you can even successfully stretch a troubled muscle group. Your nervous system must create new firing orders and sequences when we have poorly balanced postures. Nerves run through muscles and if the muscle is shut down, then its signal strength is compromised to.

For example: Someone is experiencing front shoulder pain. Most would stretch the pec and strengthen the posterior shoulder with lats (latissimus dorsi/back). However, it is very possible that your pecs are tight and are not able to stretch because the of the way that our bodies have wound themselves up. Typically, the biceps become the muscles that experience constant firing (just like hip flexors) and become very tight. Remember what we said about muscle groups?

If one is short, then the other is long, and the rest of the body will adapt accordingly. We must lengthen the biceps to restore balance back in that pair, plus its affected neighbors. The only way to successfully stretch a muscle is under its own tension. We must repeatedly stretch the biceps eccentrically, so they can lengthen, release tension in the group, and as well as throughout the chain. Furthermore, we must also remember that it may not just be the biceps. Our hip tension effects our ribcage and the musculature. It is quite possible that it is our hip musculature that is keeping the rib cage rotated, thus forcing the shoulder to stay internally rotated, and will also keep the posterior muscle shut down. I have seen countless internally rotated shoulders release and lay flat on the table just by stretching the biceps. It was also the key muscle group that was part of my shoulder recovery and I can tell you that the release is magical.

Remember, it's not just a matter of front to back, or one opposing muscle to another. Each muscle has some relationship (either directly or indirectly) with another. Furthermore, the internal musculature adjusts as well. This systematic way of work is also capable of lengthening the internal core. Your body is the Divinely designed machine that we call our body. It is supposed to do this. Some of those reasons are because situations occur in our daily lives require it to;

1. Keep our postural alignment where we demand it to be at any instant.
2. Under duress, muscles call upon neighboring muscles to assist so that your body can successfully complete a movement. We call this muscle compensation.
3. During extreme overload another muscle a muscle can fail completely and needs another to do its job. (substitution).

The idea of core training is to turn on the weakened and inactive "core muscles." A great and mandatory approach to all exercise. Over time these muscles weaken and lead to changes of strength and stability throughout the body.

Let's take another perspective regarding core muscles. The rule of thumb is, "if any muscle is not working or is weak, then something else is doing its job." Well, what if we approached the compensating muscles that are shutting down the weak muscles first? If we corrected those muscles, then what would happen? They would change the way that our body is aligned, firing, and sending information in the musculature. It would send more responsibility back to the muscles that were being substituted or compensated for. Turning on the core requires not just excessive stimulation, it requires our muscles to become more sequentially balanced out so that the core can fire all on its own. Shut down muscles are not getting nervous system information because it is being diverted to other muscles. We must unravel the entire musculature if we want to restore the core. The core is our structural foundation and its center is the starting point of all movement. If we don't fully restore length and tension, then the core will never perform at its best. Furthermore, if it is compromised, then building on top of it will likely lead to more compensating patterns and inevitable breakdown.

We must fully restore the muscles including the deep core muscles. This is the first step at improving overall efficiency. Once this happens, then the rest of the body changes its calibration, and we can improve the way that we train any muscle. It happens 10 times faster and with less intense effort as well. This work will restore the length/tension relationship in the body back to as close to as 50/50 as possible. This is how we can achieve true neuromuscular efficiency. This is how pain disappears and it works on your novice client up to your ELITE athlete.

The Most Important Rules of Training
SAFETY, SAFETY, SAFETY!!

Let's first define what safety is in the context of exercise:
1. Careful examination of important life diagnostics (eg. Blood-pressure, resting heart rate etc.)
2. Through examination of movement and physical well-being
3. Not doing ANYTHING that compromises #1 & #2!

We briefly spoke about neuro-muscular efficiency in the previous chapters and its role in our physiology. Now I would like to talk about how it is THE MOST important entity in any exercise program and how it matters ALL OF THE TIME!

This system will show you how we can easily install exercises and techniques that will rapidly increase anyone's neuromuscular efficiency. Furthermore, it will provide the answer to the question, "what is the most effective way to train a client."

The body has all the answers that it needs, sometimes it just needs help to see them. That is our job as Fitness/Personal Trainers and with this system, we will have them available always.

The Muscular Re-Calibration System (MRS) is designed to assess kinetic chain breakdowns, muscle compensation patterns, and gives you the precise programming to correct it for any training program by using eccentric based muscle stretching. The results are immediate, profound, and vital for the evolution of Fitness programming.

Below are some details about the MRS

Primary Focus: To assess, survey, and repair Kinetic chain breakdown in exercise by using a simplified, universal Mobility system that is combined with eccentric muscle stretching.

"Muscular Re-Calibration System" uses three basic exercises to assess muscle group balance and synergy at all 5 Kinetic checkpoints. These three exercises are the overhead squat, plank, and push-up. The scores for each of these exercises have a designated correction and reinforcement program to follow.

Content of the Program and How is it Identified: The program materials consist of a Universal Mobility Assessment scoring sheet, Muscular Re-Calibration Solutions guide, and a Muscular Re-Calibration Reinforcement training program.

Program Oversight: Participants will begin with a brief kinesiology review with an in-depth look at muscle group imbalances and how these imbalances create a cumulative effect in our musculature. Fitness professionals already know a lot of other important principles about the body. The language and design of this system is to help them re-arrange the information that they already know and use it specifically to change the body before they begin strengthening it. Personal Trainers/Fitness professionals already have an extensive understanding of how the body works using concentric muscle contraction. As their focus shifts to only programing for eccentric repetitions, it will help them to create a greater success when bringing us back to efficiency, thus significantly improving their client's exercise results.

Your client will be assessed using three basic exercises. Those exercises are the Overhead Squat, the Plank, and the Push-up. Each exercise score from 0 to 5. Each number has its own precise instructions on the Muscular Re-Calibration Answer Key that will improve the client's mobility almost immediately. Furthermore, it explains why a movement is occurring that way and gives further suggestions to help move the client along in their training.

There are two different release sequences, release Sequence 1 for the lower body, and release Sequence 2 for the upper body. Both sequences follow a precise pattern that will allow the practitioner to re-calibrate the body through exercise. These exercises will target the tightest muscles of the group first.

The reinforcement exercises are paired in sequence to strengthen the weak muscle groups and to re-train the nervous system, so it properly performs the desired movement without any muscle compensations occurring.

The MRS was designed to identify improper body mechanics and to provide solution for any imbalance no matter how complicated the problems are. It can be understood by anyone with a Valid, Nationally Accredited Personal Trainer certification and/or a background in exercise science. It provides masterful, corrective exercise solutions written in an easy to follow exercise program. Basically, if you understand how to program exercise, then you can use these sequences to receive great results with any client.

The Muscular Re-calibration system is the link between true neuro-musculo-skeletal efficiency and exercise. We have spent decades incorporating many great techniques that will improve most people's posture, strength, and overall physique. Many of these tactics have had great success as well. However, by applying eccentric phase muscle stretching as a matter of mandatory programming we fulfill a necessary need that traditional programming misses. The MRS is measurable, easily interpreted, and can be applied universally across any human being.

We are the perfect machine with many perfected processes. The more that we understand the body for what it is, then the more that we can have the body do what we want it to do. It is designed to adjust to its environment regardless of modern architecture, footwear, and other external influences. The body has the leverage to instantaneously create a new state for itself as needed. However, once it becomes over-leveraged, then that's when things will go wrong.

The body will learn whatever you teach it. Teach it through careful balanced programming and not by force. Re-calibrate the body in a manner that it can function as efficient as possible and watch your body come to life!

Typical Pain Troubleshooting

You say that you are experiencing pain somewhere. Maybe it's your lower back? Well, this didn't happen overnight. The muscles in your thighs, hips, glutes, and even your shoulders have been over-leveraged for quite some time. Now, it's showing up in your back. We are also all one-side dominant creatures. That means that we have a favorite side. Most people are right side dominant (although it can be argued that we are lefty's in a right-handed world). Our natural body rotation between our torso towards our hips goes from left to right and right to left as we move. It's a constant mechanical function of our bodies and a likely predictor of how our bodies will adjust over time.

As righties move, they begin by reaching from right to left. The dominant movement in the lower body is the opposing foot, because it counters the reaching upper body. Regardless of which side dominance you are, the rotation and calibration almost always follow the dominantly used side. However, if there is a dominant activity or incident (such as an accident) that favored a change in side dominance, then the body will adjust accordingly. Furthermore, any context that changes your dominant firing patterns are built on top of your original movement patterns. The newer adjustments hide the initial foundation adjustments and force the body to move in ways that it is not capable of sustaining for a long period of time. This is another reason injuries can become complicated.

These changes will show up in real time every day and with every movement. Now, because of the extreme overleveraging in your body, wear and tear becomes more constant. Basically, your body is being torn up every time that you move. Imagine a twisted towel that starts twisting the opposite direction except it does so without unwinding. Now imagine your body doing the same. OWWWW!!!!

As a muscle changes its length, every other muscle in the body is affected by it, and it must adjust. They are programmed and designed that way. Moreover, every single system in the body integrates with another just as the nervous, muscular, and skeletal system do. Out of the 10 major systems in the body, not 1 is left to work alone. Every single major system will affect another. If one becomes weak or compromised, then it is likely another is overactive (however not always the case). If the network is slow or shut down, then it can weaken all processes in the body.

The Reality of Your Body

Now, what does this all mean? It means that the body has a pattern and a purpose. It means that everything that occurs in our body is based from systematic programming and not symptomatic. If we significantly overuse one muscle, then the rest of the body systematically changes to support it. The body is constantly communicating with itself. It signals when the system is not working correctly. Usually this is what pain is for. It's not a punishment although at times it can feel depressingly horrific. It just had to scream at us, so we would finally pay attention. If we ignore these symptoms, they won't just go away, and only addressing symptoms will not restore the system.

Our bodies go through incredible bouts of movement, breakdown, exertion, and abuse. It's an absolute that our bodies will go through this. They were designed for those reasons. The body is constantly repairing and recycling itself. A problem in one place is NEVER about a single occurrence unless something caused isolated trauma to it such as an IMPACT. An event such as a car accident or fall can also be a trigger for an injury however, your body's ability to absorb the shock created during the accident may play a role in how much it will affect you. Remember, the body is ready for anything unless it's being distracted by something else.

Your Network is Criss-Crossed

All information systems have a specific way of delivering messages and our body is the most sophisticated system on Earth. It is designed to make instantaneous adjustments when the primary channel is compromised. Consider how many systems mirror the human body and work with high efficiency. The internet for example is what we refer to as, "the information super-highway." It can send trillions of bits of information per second to anywhere on Earth (even in space). It too can have loading issues or slowed connection. During the times when there is interference in the primary channel, a secondary network can be used. It could be weaker and/or slower, however, it still manages to get the messages through eventually. At the end of the day, we typically only care about one thing, sending our message and we don't really care how it gets there.

The body is no different. If the fastest route is not getting the messages through fast enough (or at all), then it sends it through alternative routes. They may be weaker, slower, or just plain inappropriate, however, they still must find a way to get the message delivered. Have you ever seen a hunched back old man with a cane walking, leaning to one side, and is barely upright enough crossing the street? Well, he's still walking, right?! The brain NEVER forgets. It always will find a way to get it done even if it is done in a highly undesired way. It is systematically PERFECT. Yes, it's perfect even when it's not operating efficiently it still create a balance somehow even if it's in an ass-backwards way.

We all commit to a level of discomfort before we decide to correct pain (if at all). We learned at an early age that the body heals itself. We also learned that the body slows down as we age so we accept that aches and pains are part of the aging process. Well, let's change perspectives for a second:

It is an absolute fact that our DNA does replicate slower as we age. Moreover, it is also a fact that over time we wear out our bodies as we age. We lose muscle, our balance can suffer, and it becomes tougher to move. We can dramatically improve that if we just restore neuro-musculo-skeletal efficiency. We can essentially, "turn back the hands of time" just by restoring these connections in the older population. Weak signals lead to decreased mobility, strength, energy, balance, flexibility, and more. Restoring the systems in the older population will help them to restore natural strength, body mechanics, power, healing, and allow greater overall function within their bodies.

Client Case Studies

Case #1- Jill S: Injury included 2 knee surgeries (1 total re-construct), lack of sensation in the quadriceps muscle group on the injured leg (via touch or physical reflex), limping, very minimal range of motion in her right knee, and constant pain.

Assessment: Upon my initial assessment, I visually noticed out of balanced hips. Her score on the Universal Mobility Analysis scored her a 0 due to pain and her inability to initiate her hips backwards was not possible. After muscle testing, I found that her left posterior pelvic muscles were extremely tight at the spine and in the lower back.

Her left side was significantly overstimulated due to injury compensation. This created an over stimulation in her left adductor muscles, psoas, lower back, and tension in the right groin muscle.

This over-leveraging of her musculature prior to her injury and the time after her treatment were keeping her hips locked in a position where her quad muscles were shut down. Furthermore, there was an enormous amount of scar tissue surrounding her knee where the trauma and procedure took place.

Jill's preliminary prognosis from her Surgeon and PT: The nerves leading to the quadriceps muscles were damaged during the injury and the surgery. She was told that nothing more could be done for her. She should accept that she will never run again and consider moving to a warmer climate. Furthermore, she was categorized as "permanently disabled."

During our initial session, I began unwinding the dominant muscles that were keeping her hips locked into place. After 60 minutes, she had slightly more knee flexion and she stopped limping.

As we continued our work she improved significantly with each session. Increasingly more scar tissue began to break up due to her improved range of motion, her pain began to go down, and sensation returned to her quadriceps muscles.

By 4 sessions she was no longer in pain and confident that she would make a full recovery.

Session 9: I watched carefully as Jill could run on a treadmill for ¼ of a mile without pain.

Session 10: Jill scored a 4 out of 5 on the Universal Mobility Analysis and could successfully run half of a mile on a treadmill without pain.

Session 12 was a post-race adjustment after her 1st 5 k run since her surgery.

Conclusion and Summary:

Jill had begun her Fitness journey to become healthier. As she began running, her body already had a set calibration that did not promote excessive running. Her job and lifestyle also were an influencing variable. She was a Nurse (a physically demanding job) and overweight (70 + lbs. lost). Her lifestyle alone was enough to create over-leveraging in her body. Once she added in exercise that her body was not prepared to handle, then her body improper mechanics created a problem at her knee. Furthermore, I found out that her lower back tightness was present before any of her knee issues. This already indicates a calibration problem. The addition of running and exercise placed even greater demand on her body that it was not prepared to do. The result was that her knee suffered and failed.

Her knee was never the problem, it was just a symptom. All of her lifelong movement patterns caused her to run improperly thus, damaging her knee.

Our work together allowed me to trace backwards joint by joint and to reset her entire body's musculature. As a result, her muscles, bones, joints, and nervous system were communicating properly. Her strength returned, her pain disappeared, and she could get her lifestyle back.

Case #2- : Michael- Injury: Michael had suffered from crushed vertebrae during a work accident 12 years prior to our work. He had several disc procedures which included the removal of his L4-L5 vertebrae. Michael came to me because of left knee problems. The pain in his left knee led to two procedures to relieve the pain in his knee.

My initial opinion was that his hip alignment from his lower back injury was leading to restricted hip joint movement and excessive tension at the knee.

My physical observation of his squat scored him a 0 on the Muscular Re-Calibration System. He could not initially move his hips back and without pain. He also had not been able to touch his toes in nearly 20 years.

Through muscle testing I found what I suspected. His deep internal core and lower back muscles were holding his hips tightly to his spine. His quads had little response to muscle testing, his inner thighs, and groin were extremely tight, and his lower back was nearly ceased up.

As your hips become tight and your lower back becomes compressed, the femur will become tighter in the hip socket. Extremely tight hip musculature will stop the proper ball and socket rotation in the hips. The body then looks for the next link in the kinetic chain to provide movement, in this case the knee.

Our treatment began at the knee. Due to the sensitivity of both the knee and the spine I worked at improving his range of motion in his hip joints, then his knees. My end goal was to create more freedom at this spine to stop the constant knee flares while providing maximal restoration of his spine flexibility.

Michael and I worked 2 hours during our first session (this is not typical but can be necessary in some extreme cases). We had to unwind him both in his lower and upper body. The result of our first sessions brought him instant knee relief. Due to his professional travel schedule we met for our second session 1 month later.

Sessions 2 was also 2 hours because he needed a lot of attention to both upper and lower body. However, after our 2nd session, Michael's squat range of motion immediately improved to a 3 out of 5 (90 degree squats without pain). Furthermore, Michael could touch his toes for the first time in 20 years.

Conclusion and Summary

Both of Michael's injuries came from improper function in his neuro-musculo-skeletal system. His work in construction placed so much demand on his body that his muscles created extreme trauma at his spine. The procedure to correct the symptoms merely reduced the symptoms and their severity. The problem that created his back pain was a total body systematic failure. His lifestyle after his back procedure stripped him of his livelihood and caused him to move with extreme caution to avoid re-injuring himself. After 12 years of compensated movements the knee issue arose from his confused body.

Michael will always live with a missing vertebra and will have to take caution in activities the that he does to protect it. However, since our work he can drastically strengthen his core muscle. This helped him to keep out of pain, improve the structural integrity of his body, and gave him his ability to move free of flare ups.

At the time Michael was 42 years old. Prior to our work his prognosis was the continue seeing further degeneration of his body and as he aged they predicted him to need walking assistance in his early 60's. Instead, he went back to work and now enjoys a life with minimal to no interruption. Muscular Re-Calibration restored his systems to as optimal as possible. Now he is free to live his life and not suffer from it.

Special Case Study: Parkinson's Disease

Dan E: – My work with Dan has been one of the most rewarding experiences of my life. Dan began working with me because he wanted to relieve pain associated with his inactivity and illness. What I discovered changed my understanding of the body forever in a profound way.

Dan had a very aggressive form of Parkinson's. He was diagnosed 18 months before we met and was already having significant complications. He lost his ability to walk unassisted, had a urostomy bag for his urine, significant dementia, and pain in his lower/mid back. However, there was one thing that Parkinson's did not take from him and that was his spirit.

Dan was a fighter and an optimist. His goal wasn't just to feel comfortable, it was to get his body back. He always used to say, "When I get back to doing the weights it will be a great day." I was always willing to take on extreme cases. I knew that I could help in some way but, the rate of success that could be attained in his case was unknown to me at the time. I saw results with another client with Parkinson's disease a couple of years prior to meeting Dan, so I knew that I could help a bit. The difference this time is that I spent 6 months working with Dan twice a week and the results were shocking.

As I first began to work with Dan a few things changed right away. His balance got immediately better, some pain started to fade, and his voice began to deepen. People that have Parkinson's can experience a shallower sounding voice. It losses its depth because of the weakened diaphragm, jaw, and throat muscles. This happened within his first 2 sessions. Although his body still had Parkinson's disease, it began to restore more sharpness as we worked. Session after session he improved. His tremors decreased in their intensity or stopped all together. Eventually after 3 months I finally got him back to a workout.

We kept it easy and put him on some machines. He was so happy to be back at the weights. Let me tell you this guy knew his stuff too. We would talk about form and exercise science often. He used to tell me how back in the day he used to work out with the guys that started it all back in Venice Beach. Dan was also a Navy man, so he was always in great physical shape. I remember him telling me about how someone approached him about his form doing a triceps workout once. His reply to the guy was, "If Lou Ferrigno tells you to do it that way, then that's how you do it." He always had humor and spunk. I was working with a man that never quit and was always doing what he loved.

Things started going downhill for Dan shortly thereafter fast. He was in and out of the hospital with infections almost weekly, but I would still visit his home to keep his muscles loose and his body feeling more alive. As Dan's condition began to worsen other things started fading. However, no matter how bad things got, his body ALWAYS responded to our work. Although his neurological control was quickly fading, his brain always accepted our work together. That is a profound finding!

Not once did his brain forget how to work. It just weakened in its ability to control the signals and deliver them. It always responded and adapted accordingly. Even on home hospice I performed this work on him. It was an honor to be there for him when he heeded help the most and a blessing to see what the body is truly capable of.

We are often given a condition or classified into a category when we experience illness or injury. It is very easy to fall into a doomed mindset when trouble arises. My work with Dan proved to me that not only can I help the injured, but I could help ANYONE. Our work together inspired me to work closely with those that had Parkinson's disease for the next couple of years. They were not as ill as Dan and had even greater results. This work stopped their tremors, improved balance issues, and progressed their bodies back to full activity! Some were not even able to sit up without assistance and began walking without a walker.

It is incredible!

I share Dan's story because it sets such a huge precedent. The marvel of this work is how effectively we can communicate with the nervous system and ask it to change what it knows. It inspired me to work with as many new conditions as possible and ALL had very similar results. I've worked with so many people that were told by leading experts that there was nothing that can be done for their situation and this worked was the treatment that helped them.

We are on the leading edge of the next age of physiology and healing. It is my goal to change the text books and the perspectives of every professional that works with a physical modality. This is how the body works, period. We no longer need to look around for patch work or cover-up solutions like pain meds. Surgeries can be significantly decreased and avoided altogether. People can live fulfilled lives rather than suffer. We are all capable of receiving this type of treatment and programming. The body always knows what to do, it just got side-tracked and needs to be re-calibrated. That is what I do for others and you can too.

APPENDIX A
<u>UNIVERSAL MOBILITY ANALYSIS</u>

Objective: To identify kinetic chain/posture breakdown the client and apply the required Mobility therapy program

The Assessment:

1. ***Overhead Squat***: The overhead squat assesses sequential upper and lower body range of motion. (5 points)

Stand up straight with feet hips to shoulder width apart and hands at your side. Using a dowel, place it on your head while holding it w your arms at a 90 –degree angle. Lower the bar to your shoulders. Initiate the hips backwards and down while raising the arms + bar straight over your head. The end range will be when a full squat is achieved and the arms are behind the head in a locked position (shoulder blades down and together). The goal is to sit in a full squat with arms extended over and behind the head. Score your exercise by using the answer key below.

- 0– Pain
- 1– Cannot initiate hips back, or fully extend arms overhead
- 2– Can initiate hips back, some scapular retraction, and can reach ¼ depth squat with stable knees
- 3– Achieved 90 degrees squat with full scapular retraction and elbow extension (no deviation in knees or elbows)
- 4– At ¾'s depth with little or no scapular retraction
- 5– Full Squat with full retraction (all joints are in line and stable)

2. ***Plank:*** The plank will measure the level of upper/lower body stability and synergy (5 points)

Bring the client to the floor onto their hands and knees. If this is not achievable then find an elevated surface such as a bench. If on the floor, have the client maintain a 90 degree bent elbow with their forearms on the floor. Then, have them straighten their legs and straighten their hips. They must be able to squeeze the abs, quads, and glutes at the same time (If they clearly are incapable of using a straight leg plank, then switch to bent knee). They should be able to maintain the contraction of the shoulder blades at the same time as they are contracting the lower body. They should resemble a long body like a "plank" of wood. Record as follows:

- 0- Pain
- 1- Cannot initiate hip extension at any level
- 2- Can initiate full hip extension but no scapular retraction
- 3- Can simultaneously reach sequential core firing and scapular retraction from a modified position
- 4- Can reach hip, leg extension, but cannot initiate scapular retraction
- 5- Full Plank achieved (full hip, leg extension, and scapular retraction

3.   ***The Push-up:*** This test will assess the clients' neuromuscular synergy while under resistance (5 points)

Have the client begin again at the same level as the plank (elevated, modified, or regular). Have the arms straight down with the hands spaced at shoulder width or wider. Keep the hands and elbows positioned at mid chest, keeping the shoulder blades slightly contracted. Have the client lower their bodies down by hinging open from the front shoulders, bringing the bent elbows/shoulder blades back to 90 degrees. All of the core muscles must be fully engaged through the entire movement. Record your observations as follows

- 0- Cannot get onto the floor or pain
- 1- Cannot initiate hip extension and/or scapular retraction/depression at any level
- 2- Can initiate hip extension and scapular retraction/depression from a modified position but not simultaneously
- 3- Synergistic hip extension and scapular retraction in any modified position
- 4- Can initiate full loaded, straight arm push-up position
- 5- Can perform at least one push-up (½ to full depth) while maintaining scapular retraction/depression and sequential core activation

APPENDIX B
Muscular Re-Calibration System Solutions Guide

Mobility and Posture Assessment #1
Client Troubleshooting and Programming

Overhead Squat Score ______

0- Client Experiences Pain

Solution: Refer back to Pre-screening assessment. If the client has not been cleared for exercise, then seek a Dr.'s approval. If client has been cleared for exercise then we select a more appropriate squatting exercise.

Suggested Trouble Shooting and Programming: Supported squat (hands on table, a bar, or by using a TRX). If pain still exist then foam rolling, stretching, and muscle rebalancing techniques must be introduced.

Follow release sequence #1 for locked hips

1- Cannot initiate hips back or overhead extension of the arms

Recommended Therapies: Practice hip flexion exercises with support (TRX, Hand supported)

Overhead Extension- Visually Assess the overhead extension of the arms/shoulder. Note the joint movements that are locked and program to strengthen their balancing (opposing) muscle.

Recommended Therapies: Shoulder Integrity Exercises, reintroduce the opposite movements to the overused parts of the body (ex. Scapular retraction/depression to counter elevation and protraction) in a 2:1 ratio)

Further Troubleshooting: See *Release Sequence 1* for hips, and *Release Sequence 2* for shoulders.

Client Scores **2-5**: Apply both corrective sequences 1 &2 in the appropriate areas to increase ROM

Mobility and Posture Assessment #2
Client Troubleshooting and Programming

Plank Score________________

0- Client experiences Pain or cannot get onto the floor

Solution: If client has been cleared at pre-screening, then take the appropriate actions as follows

-For elderly or diminished capacity clients ask them to plank on a high surface. If that still is not possible, then eliminate this test.

-If the client experiences pain, then regress the exercise. If pain still exists, then stop the test. Refer to appropriate Mobility Therapy that corresponds to location of the pain/discomfort.

1- Client cannot initiate hip extension at any level

Recommended Therapies: Foam roll the hips, top of the quads, top of the glutes and hip complex. Follow-up with a manual stretch, and perform modified hip extension exercises. If the glutes still seem to be inhibited and hip extension does not progress, then refer to *Release Sequence #1*

2- Can initiate ¾ – full hip extension but no scapular retraction/depression

- This is a very common place for people to score because the full activation of the hip extensors will exaggerate the forward upper body posture that was compensating for the adjustments in the lower core.
- Stretch upper body or apply dynamic release techniques for shoulder complex, arms, scapulae, and follow up with movement reinforcing exercises
- If the client does not respond to any therapies, then see *Release Sequence #2*

Mobility and Posture Assessment #2
Client Troubleshooting and Programming
Plank Continued:

Score 3-5: Sequential Firing of core muscles and upper body brings the spine into neutral

-Select appropriate level of exercise based on the clients' ability to do it (min 10 seconds/max 30)

Apply both *Release Sequence 1 & 2* as needed to progress their strength and ability.

Follow reinforcement strategies as needed in the clients' workouts.

Mobility and Posture Assessment #3
Client Troubleshooting and Programming
Push-up Score________

0- Client has pain or cannot get onto the floor

If the client cannot get on the floor have them place their hands on an elevated surface such as a bar, plyo box, or even a counter top. Ask them to perform a push up. If this still is inappropriate for the client, then place them in a chair and have them perform the unloaded movement of a pushup with hands and elbows at the nipple line. If the client still cannot do this for any reason, then eliminate the test and refer to *Release Sequence #2*

If client can achieve a push-up then use the next scores to break down their movement.

1- Cannot initiate hip extension, scapular retraction/depression at any level of difficulty.

   See troubleshooting for plank scores of: **1 & 2,** or eliminate the test.

2- Can initiate hip extension and scapular retraction/depression from a modified position but not simultaneously

   Apply ***Release Sequences 1 & 2*** and use the plank reinforcement strategies **<u>until sequential firing of the upper and lower body is achieved.</u>**
   Recommended progressions: Follow reinforcement strategies for plank plus strengthen the main muscle groups involved (core, triceps, posterior deltoid, & chest) in order to progress to ***#3.***

3- Synergistic hip extension and scapular retraction in any modified   position

   Continue to improve muscle group balance and synergy until the client can complete 10 perfect reps at modified position.

4- Can initiate full loaded, straight arm push-up position
   Have the client perform a push-up and record their depth. If fully dept is not achieved for at least 1 push-up then use the Shoulder Girdle

reinforcement Program Accordingly until the client re-tests at full depth

5- Push-up achieved at full depth
Continue to apply Upper and Lower Body Reinforcement strategies in your client's workouts several times a week.

Appendix C Muscular Re-calibration Sequences
Re-Calibration Sequence #1

-Lumbo-pelvic-hip Complex
Stretching and Rebalancing with Eccentric Reps
The most important concept of this stretch is to maintain a constant contraction on the target muscle and to maintain a slow 10 second eccentric phase with each rep. Note: all movements must initially begin with a 2 second isometric contraction on the first rep
Each set is 90 seconds long (60 seconds or less for weaker clients)
All exercises should perform 5 regular strength training reps before applying stretch sets
We want the client to begin with a 1 second concentric rep, 2 second Isometric contraction, maintain a steady tension on the target muscle, and slowly release the target muscle for 10 a second eccentric rep count. Repeat with a 1:2:10 concentric/isometric/eccentric rep count.

(note: do not let the clients fight back or increase the tension in the target muscle while eccentrically stretching or the stretch will stop. If this happens then just reset, start a new rep and continue the set.

Trouble Shooting for Hip Imbalances

Muscle Groups must be stretched in the written order. If pain or discomfort appears at any point in the rep range, then that muscle's rep range ends at the site of discomfort. Repeat the sequences until discomfort disappears and range of motion increases.

1. **Hamstrings/Quadriceps:** *With Machines–* Alternate leg curls/leg extensions by using a leg curl machine and leg extension machine. (Weighted Resistance should be at a 50% 1 RM) Formula: 1 second concentric. 2 second isometric, 10 seconds concentric, and repeat

   Without machines– Hamstrings stretching can be done from a seated (easiest) or supine position (more complex). Start: have your client engage hips/abdominal muscles, then bend their knee for a hamstring contraction. With a band, pull against the leg and begin straightening it over a 10 second count. Use the same rep count as a machine based set, then repeat on the opposite leg.

   Note Each rep is a 1:2:10 concentric/isometric/eccentric count.

Target Muscle Start: Hamstring

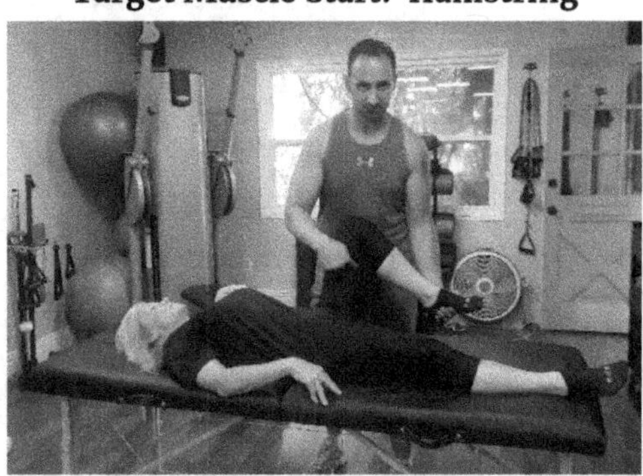

Target Muscle End: Hamstrings

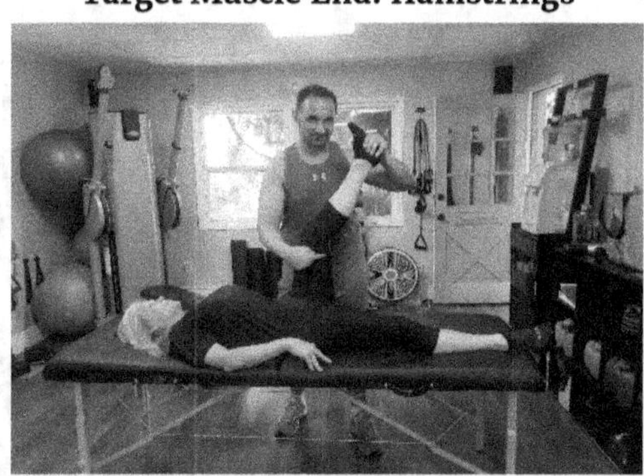

Quad Stretching can be done by doing an eccentric standing squat 1:2:10 concentric/isometric/eccentric rep count (use assist if needed) all while maintaining a constant hold on the quads.

Continue this sequence by alternating between balancing muscle groups (hamstring/quads) and repeat this for 4-6 sets.

*For clients with limited mobility have them sit in a chair and use a resistance band. Loop the band around the front of their legs (lower tibialis) near the top of the ankle and you hold resistance against their legs. Have them extend their legs and you pull their legs slowly back into knee flexion.

Continue this sequence by alternating between balancing muscle groups (hamstring/quads) and repeat this for 2-3 sets until the client scores higher on the assessment.

Target Muscle Begin: Quadriceps

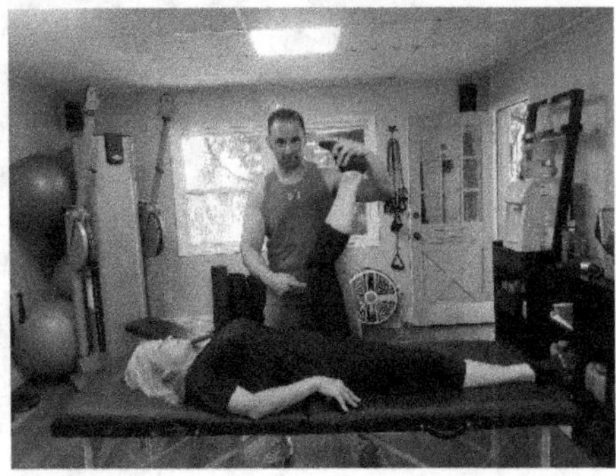

Target Muscle End: Quadriceps

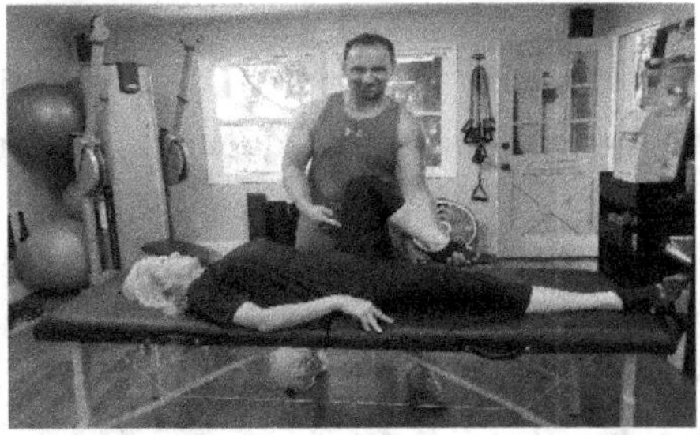

2. **Hip Flexors:** Using Abdominal machines
(Weighted Resistance should be at 50-60% 1 RM)

Using Machines: Abdominal Machines with lower abdominal portions for hip flexor stretch – Have your clients engage their lower abdominals by concentrating on raising the knees towards their chest.). We want the client to do a 2 second Isometric contraction after the concentric phase, maintain a steady hold and slowly release the abdominals for a 10 second eccentric rep count. Repeat the rep with a 1:2:10 concentric/isometric/eccentric count.

Hip flexor stretch without equipment. Have the client lie on their backs on a bench with their hands under their hips for added stability. Keep their hips at the edge of the bench with their feet aimed at the ground. Have them bring their knees back to their chest as far as possible by using their hip flexors and keeping their legs bent for a 1 second count, hold the pose for 2, then slowly release the front of their hips and lower their feet towards the ground for a 10 second count. Draw the knees back on a 1 second concentric phase and repeat 4-6 sets.

sequential firing of the glutes, quads, and rear upper back muscles, then the stretch has stopped. Have the client return to the start position and repeats the exercise.

Stretch accordingly for 4-6 sets

Target Muscle Begin: Hip Flexor

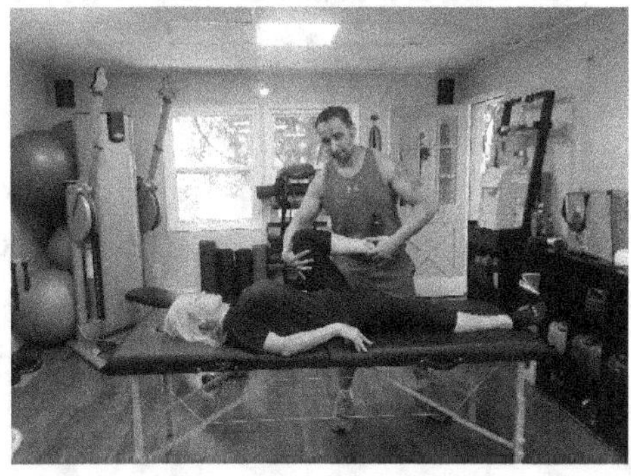

Target Muscle End: Hip Flexor

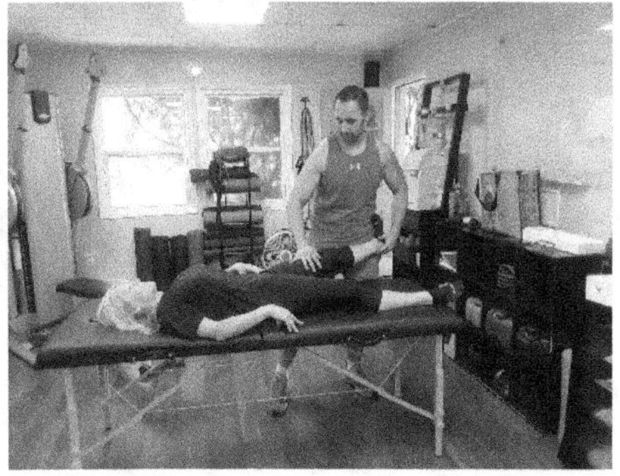

3. Inner/Outer Thighs

(Weighted Resistance should be at 50-60% 1 RM)

Alternate add/abduction with the inner outer thigh machine.

Inner Thigh: Have the client to do a 1 second hip adduction concentric contraction, a 2 second isometric contraction, and a slow 10 second eccentric rep count.

Outer thigh: Have the client to do a 1 second hip abduction concentric contraction, a 2 second isometric contraction, and a slow 10 second eccentric rep count.

Without Equipment: This technique requires that the trainer be hands on. The trainer will conduct a *Manual Eccentric Stretch* on the client. This requires a precise positioning, feel of muscle tension, and communication by the trainer.

Inner Thighs: Client will have to lie flat on their back with knee bent at 90 degrees and held together by their own resistance. Here the trainer will act as the machine by placing their hands against the inside of their knees. The client will then press against the trainer's hands by using their inner thighs (trainer does not have to give 100% of their strength but must make the client do some work) to prime the muscle connection.

Begin

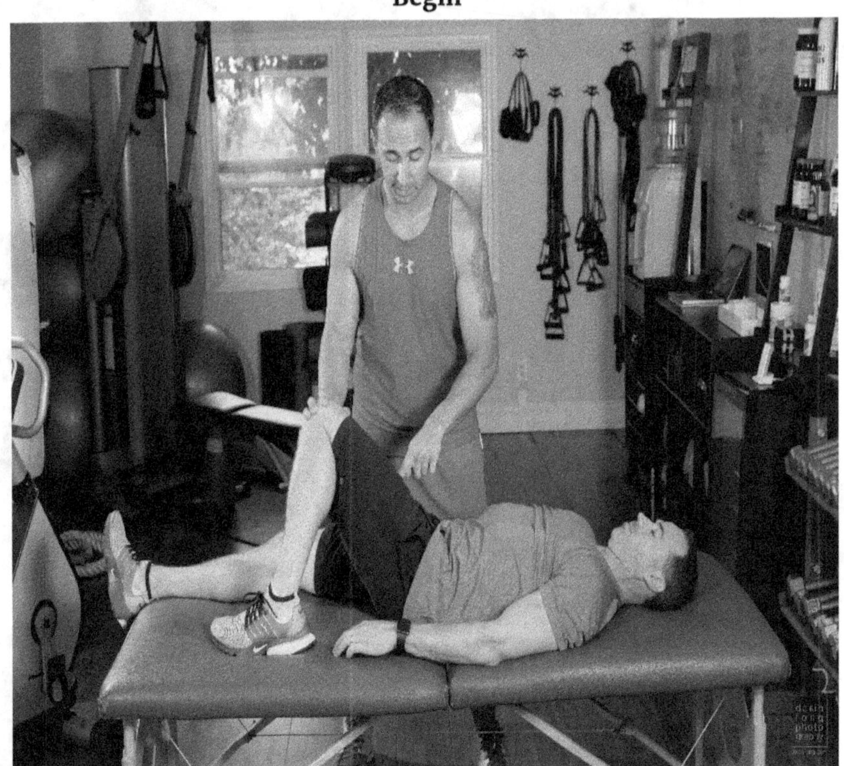

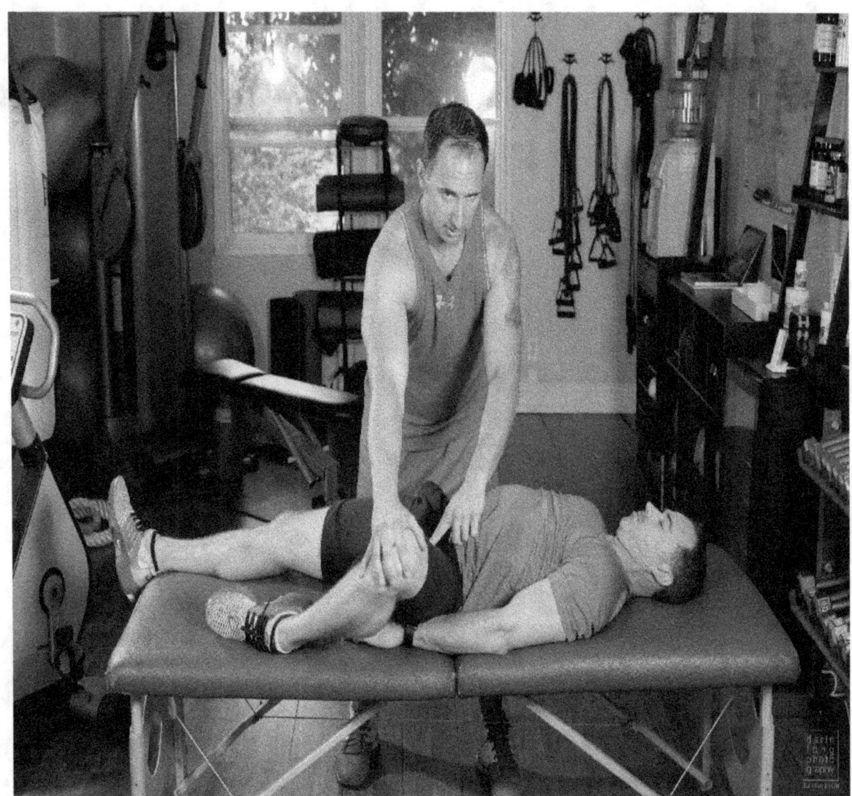

End

Next, the client must keep their knees together and the trainer must slowly open the client's knees until the body stops moving. Have the client close their legs and repeat 5-10 times. (note: this area of the body is can be very sensitive for both you and the client. The DOMS for this muscle group can be very lengthy, so use your best judgment when choosing the number of reps/sets for your clients).

Switch sides and repeat
Stretch accordingly for 4-6 sets

Outer thighs: The trainer should carefully position themselves perpendicular to the client so that the client's knee lines up next to the trainer's abdomen. Next instruct them to bring the knee down towards the floor as far as possible.

Once they have reached their full range of Hip Abduction, have them isometrically hold the position and the trainer will then pull the outermost knee closest to their own body. This stretch will open up the abductors, external rotators, and even some of the lower back. Repeat and keep the number of reps consistent with the rep count done on the inner thighs, then switch sides. (This stretch is great for re-establishing femoral rotation at the hip and greatly reduces knee pain).

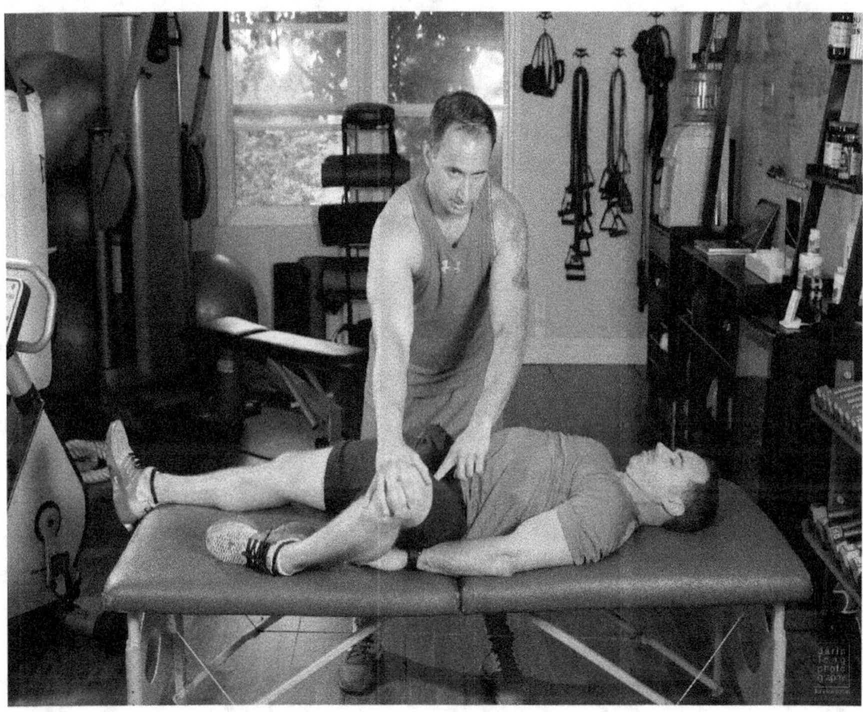

Begin

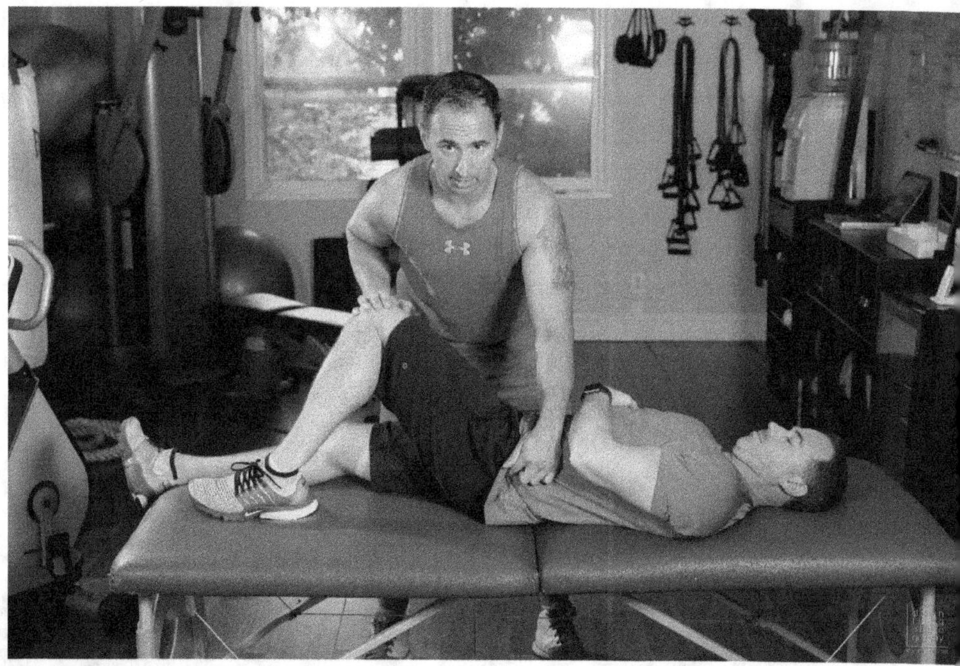

End *Switch sides and repeat*

4: Lower Back

Lower back stretch: Using a Back-extension machine, extend the lower back by keeping the quads locked (not knee just quad muscle), then engaging the glutes and lower back. Once engaged, keep the glutes and quads engaged throughout the entire concentric phase of each rep. Next, allow the torso to come forward bending at the waistline only for 10 seconds (the body will stop bending forward when its maximum stretch is reached). Extend the lower back in a 1 second count, hold for 2, slowly release it (keeping quads/glutes contracted) for 10 seconds, and repeat.

(Note: If pain occurs then, try shortening the rep range. If their pain still occurs, then go back to sequence #1). Continue this sequence by alternating between balancing muscle groups (hip flexor/lower back) and repeat this for 4-6 sets.

Lower back Stretch without machines: Light loaded stiff legged dead lifts- Give the client very light dumb bells to hold at their sides (50% 1RM or less). Also, a prone back extension chair can be used with body weight (same principles apply and only if appropriate)

While standing up straight keep the glutes/quads/lower abdominals engaged, and the rear shoulders loaded. Slowly take a bow forward and letting the dumb bells reach towards the floor (it is important to begin movement forward at the waist and not at the head). Once the back stops bending or the client loses the ability to maintain

Stretch accordingly for 4-6 sets

Re-Calibration Sequence #2

Rotator Cuff, Shoulder girdle, and Elbows
Stretching and Rebalancing with Eccentric Reps

The most important concept of this stretch is to maintain a constant contraction on the target muscle and to maintain a slow 10 second eccentric phase with each rep. Note: all movements must initially begin with a 2 second isometric contraction on the first rep

Each set is 90 seconds long (60 seconds or less for weaker clients)

4-6 sets should be performed back to back (less sets and reps for very deconditioned clients)

We want the client to begin with a 1 second concentric rep, 2 second Isometric contraction, maintain a steady tension on the target muscle, and slowly release the target muscle for 10 a second eccentric rep count. Repeat with a 1:2:10 concentric/isometric/eccentric rep count.

(note: do not fight back or increase the tension in the target muscle while eccentrically stretching or the stretch will stop. If this happens then just reset, start a new rep and continue the set.

1. **Biceps/Triceps**

    *A machine is not optimal for the test due to the general mechanics and size of my commercial gym equipment.

    Biceps curls from a seated position: Light weight dumb bell curls (40-50% 1RM)

    Begin with shoulders locked at side to avoid substitution of the deltoids (if deltoids overpower the Biceps then either lower the weight or shorten the rep range)

    Begin by holding the dumb bells with the wrists facing the midline. Bend at elbow and rotate forearm externally (outward), hold for 2 seconds, and slowly return to start position for a count of 10 (allow for internal rotation of the arm on the eccentric phase)

    Stand Triceps pushdown (using a resistance band or supine skull crushers is suitable)- Weight should be at 40-50% 1RM

    Have client engage glutes, abdominals, and thighs while in the standing position. Begin by extending the elbow and contracting the triceps, hold for two seconds, and allow for a slow return of 10 seconds. Repeat for 5-10 reps (60-90 seconds approx..) and be sure to match the number of Biceps reps.

    Again, be sure to control for substitution of deltoids and/or trapezius muscles. If pain occurs, then reduce weight, shorten rep range, or if pain still persists then get a second opinion before continuing work on these muscle groups.

    *Note- The biceps and triceps are the primary links in the chain of arm rotation. They are the main contributors of over rotation that can lead to a variety of possible rotator cuff tears. Make sure that the client is safer or aware of any damage that may already exist.

2. **Pecs and Lats-** This is where things can get a little complicated, however, if any issues with pain or range of motion are encountered, then go back to #1 Biceps/Triceps. Stretching the biceps/triceps will allow for an increase in shoulder joint range of motion.

Pecs Opener"

Lay client on back (have knees bent or place a foam roller under back of knees for increased hip stability)

Use light weight dumb bells (20-40% 1RM) This DOES NOT have to be heavy!!

Most rear deltoid muscles and mid-back muscles are totally shutdown and can only handle a marginal amount of resistance load to overload them. This is the most common mistake with most resistance training chest exercises that leads to some of the most complex muscle imbalances in the body. The overload on the anterior of the body can be devastating to the posterior chain.

Begin with arms extended, triceps fully engaged (if triceps cannot fully engage then repeat step #1 until they can), and with dumb bells in hand with wrists facing the clients lower body. Allow their arms to slowly fall backwards overhead " (note: the left side and the right side may fall into different ranges, this is ok)

Pec Opener Start

Engage pectorals(chest) and triceps, then bring the dumb bells back to the starting position, hold the contraction for 2 seconds, then slowly allow the arms to go back into the "V" position

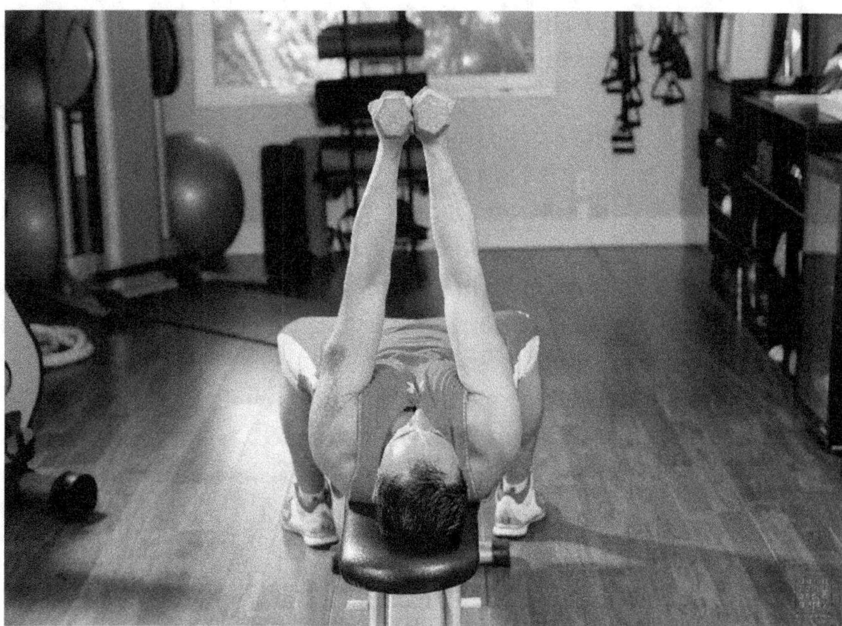

- There are three different arm rotation positions:
  1. Palms facing in (pec minor)
  2. Palms facing each other (Pec major/serratus anterior)
  3. Palms up or thumbs out (Lat and Teres Major)
     Do 10 reps for each position then repeat 4-6 times

Pec Opener End

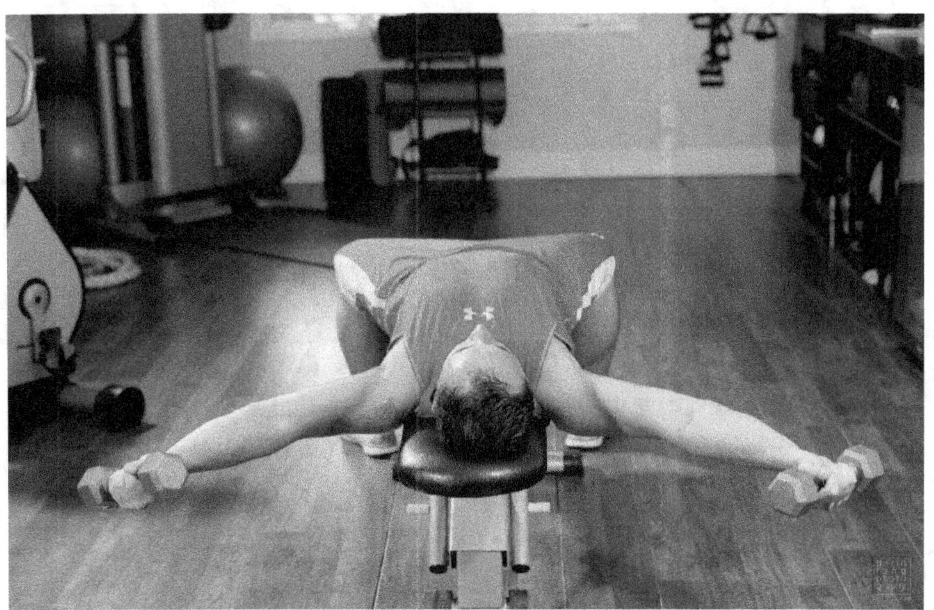

Shoulder "Clock work"

*"Clock work" will be opposite to "Pec Opener" with a couple of exceptions

"clock work" should be performed preferably from a seat position, with dumb bells (20-40% 1RM for shoulder raises) , and with slightly different hand positions (Palms up, palms down, and palms facing each other). Raise extended arms (be sure to lock the triceps) over head as far as possible without hyperextension of the lower back and/or pain into a "12 o'clock" position.

Start

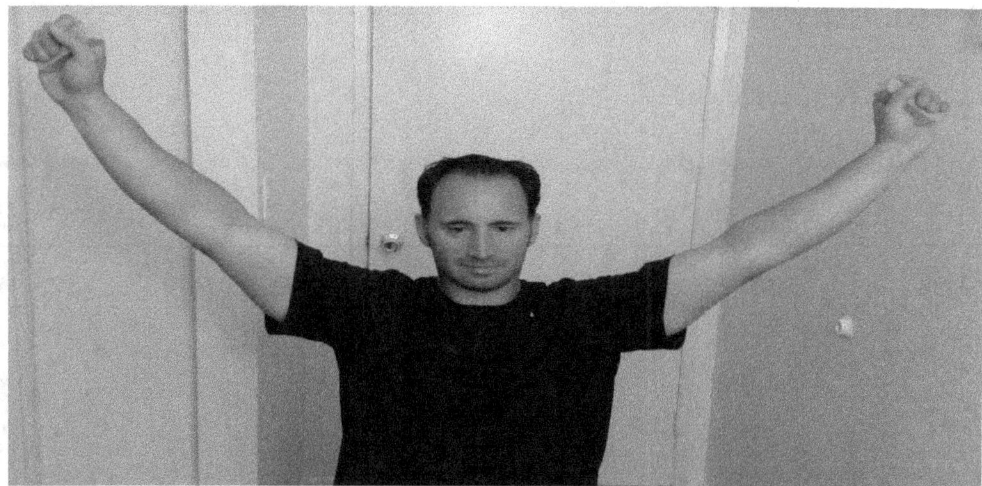

Hold the contraction in the shoulder blades, deltoids, and triceps, then slowly lower the weight back to the starting position. Repeat 5 reps for each of the 2 hand positions (palms down/ palms forward) to complete one set. Repeat 4-6 times or as needed.

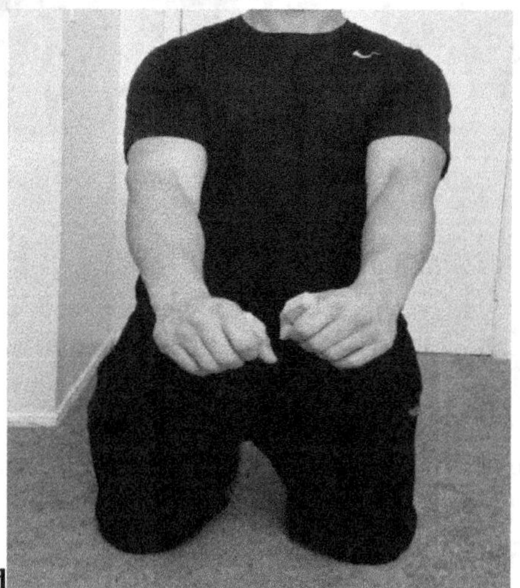

End

- If pain exists then lower weight with arms closer to the midline of the body, start from a 90-degree position, and/or return to step #1 until pain is eliminated. If pain still exists, then possible x-rays/MRI's may be needed.

5: The Neck–

There are many contributing factors regarding the neck and discomfort. The most typical of musculature imbalances include: Tight hips/psoas, intercostal muscles/pecs, and trapezius muscles. These 3 groups of muscles will promote an elevated and forward rounded shoulder girdle. This will reduce neck rotation, create pressure in the c-spine, lock up your neck muscles, and can lead to a variety of neck issues.

The most immediate decrease is in neck range of motion. This will likely cause the client to move their head by moving their shoulder girdle to replace the lost neck movement. Neck strains and disc damage are the more serious problems associated with extremely tight neck muscles.

A common misconception is that only tight traps create neck issues. The trapezius muscles will become tight because the rest of the body has created shoulder girdle elevation and these muscles are forced to stay on constantly. Furthermore, it is nearly impossible even get the bulk of the traps to stretch because the anterior chain is not giving us enough access. Remember, the traps are a posterior muscle. Without restoring the neurology to the traps by releasing the anterior chain, the will be minimal or no success at fully releasing the trapezius muscle completely.

The sequence:

1. Hip flexors, hamstrings, quads, abductors, adductors, lower back
2. Biceps, pec opener, rib cage opener (see diagram below), lats, shoulders, traps.

Repeat these sequences until lower body posture improves, rib cage releases, and traps can be stretched at full range of motion.

Further Education Opportunities:

Muscular Re-Calibration Workshops are a 2 Day, 16-hour course, and are hosted primarily at Muscle Therapy San Diego. The course provides 1.6 N.A.S.M. CEU's and should be accepted by most nationally accredited Certification Organizations.

Neil Denaut also offers 3-day, weekend mentorships for a total immersion into this system.

Please contact him for upcoming dates @muscletherapysd@gmail.com

Connect with us!

On the Web: www.muscletherapysandiego.com

Email: muscletherapysd@gmail.com

By Phone: 619-736-8995

Facebook:

https://www.facebook.com/muscletherapysandiego/